ARTHRITIS

Arthritis is a kind of catch-all condition, many complain of the symptoms which are varied enough to cover many areas of the body. In general, the major symptoms are stiffness of joints, red, inflamed and swollen joints, muscular aches and pains, deformities of the hand and foot articulations particularly, and visible bone spurs on x-ray examination. Medically speaking, there are *no known specific* causes of this disease which afflicts a minimum of 25 to 30 million Americans. Some would like to blame past infections, bad teeth, injuries, etc., for the *chronic degenerative* disease we know as arthritis.

We have purposefully emphasized the fact that specific causes are not known in so-called scientific circles and the fact that arthritis is a chronic degenerative disease. We would like to tender some evidence that all chronic degenerative disease and particularly arthritis, is due to an incomplete dietary intake of nourishing foods as close to their natural form as possible. We should understand that chronic degenerative disease is the slow, seemingly relentless deterioration of the normal structure of the body. Medical science has produced wonderful measures to control emergency disease but, by their own admission, seems powerless to halt the ravages of chronic disease.

Dr. Francis Pottenger, a well-known medical researcher, clearly established the relationship of a cooked food diet and arthritis in animals. He was able to produce arthritis at will merely by feeding cats a diet of pasteurized whole milk. Cats fed a diet of raw, whole milk had no evidence of arthritic disease whatsoever. This leads us to the obvious question: "Is the drinking of pasteurized milk the cause of arthritis?" The answer is not as simple as it may seem. Personal experience would indicate that a high percentage of arthritics are heavy consumers of pasteurized milk, ice cream, etc., but we have also observed individuals with arthritis who use very little of these products. On the other hand, in every arthritic we have ever examined or interviewed, one factor stood out, they were consuming a great majority of their food in a cooked state and had a very limited intake of raw vegetables and fruits. Often the diet consists of meat, potatoes, salad, desserts, sandwiches and processed cereals. Beverages are usually limited to coffee, tea, sugared soft drinks and alcohol.

It has, therefore, been our conclusion, by whatever degree of scientific or unscientific logic you wish to assign, that when a individual uses a predominance of *uncooked* food in his or her diet, arthritis and other degenerative diseases will not prevail in the body. A simple change to 50% raw food and 50% cooked food is often enough to prevent arthritis or to significantly alter an existing condition.

RHEUMATOID ARTHRITIS

Everyone knows that there is no effective treatment for rheumatoid arthritis. The best contributions made available by the medical establishment in the last 80 years has been the reclassification of the disease into more than 100 subdivisions. Yes, it appears as though the arthritic is hopeless. . .to be cast away like a leper. . . to hide their hands. . .to fight the pain by clenching the teeth or consuming aspirin.

The purpose of this text is to tell you something different. If you have arthritis and you do all of the things that are available, we believe that one could predict that your stiffness or pain, no matter how severe it is or how long you've had it, will or can be gone in just hours or days. . . .certainly in weeks. There are very few exceptions to this prediction. If you have the problem, it can be successfully treated. If you have the stiffness, it can be made more supple.

Here's another awesome truth. If you do not have arthritis now, you will probably have it in the future. In fact, you DO have arthritis now, even if you cannot feel it. And more than that, you give it to your children so that they will have it in the future. How much you have is only a matter of degree. Many of you can already demonstrate the presence of the disease.

WHAT IS ARTHRITIS?

There is no such thing as arthritis.

Follow me closely while I expand on this thought. There is no such thing as rheumatoid arthritis. Arthritis is a word, and a poorly defined word at that. You cannot buy it at the hardware store. You cannot get it in the mail. In fact, there are no diseases. There are just sick people.

As long as we persist in treating a word, we will go nowhere. If we treat the person, we can go somewhere. If you have a gigantic unsolvable problem, the best way to handle it is to break it down into a number of smaller solvable problems and then fix them one at a time. If we could find 50 things wrong with you and fix 40 of them, you would have to feel better.

The first step is to break the gigantic problem of arthritis down into smaller component parts.

FIRST: The anatomy of the affected area.

        Bones
        Cartilage
        Ligaments
        Connective tissues
        Muscle tissues
        Joint fluids
        Nerves
        Blood Vessels
        Lymph channels
        Geometry of function

SECOND: The physiology of the affected area.

        Arterial circulation
        Venous circulation
        Lymphatic circulation
        Sympathetic nerve flow
        Parasympathetic nerve flow
        Nutrition

Elimination
Biochemical integrity
Glandular influence

THIRD: Stress in the affected area.
Infection
Injury
Inflammation
Poisoning
Toxicity
Cellular depolarization
Permeability

Using this outline as a guide, we can begin our investigation and formulate a therapeutic plan. For example, let's take just one of the dozens of subdivisions that go under the heading of JOINT FLUIDS.

In arthritis, we must give consideration to the composition of the joint fluid because it will affect the function of the fluid.

JOINT FLUID VISCOSITY

Synovial or joint fluid is normally a sticky, viscid material with a high albumin-globulin ratio, but with an overall protein content lower than that of blood. The main constituent is mucin, which contains hyaluronic acid and chondroitin sulfate.

The hip joint contains less than one quarter teaspoon of synovial fluid. Therefore, its viscosity or thickness is very important in proper lubrication and the integrity of the joint itself. The integrity of any of the body's connective tissues depends primarily on how they are made. How much and how good is the hyaluronic acid, the chondroitin sulfate, the mucopolysaccharides and the mucoproteins? How intact are the cells that make these substances?

Of these compounds, the hyaluronic acid appears to be the substance that holds water in the tissue spaces. It holds the connective tissue cells together in a jelly-like matrix and serves as a lubricant or shock absorber in the joints. Long strands of hyaluronic acid, mixed with protein, give strength and elasticity to the connective tissue. In the joint fluid, the thickness or the viscosity depends largely on this hyaluronic acid-protein complex.

WHAT IS A DRY JOINT?

It is written that working a dry joint, a joint without sufficient lubrication even under a light load, will wear the cartilage joint covering right down to the bone is four hours. A dry joint is one that does not have enough fluid or one where the fluid has gotten too thin. In other words, the joint fluid in arthritic people is much thinner than in normal people. Therefore, it does not do its work as well or protect the joint as it should.

This is a significant statement. It could easily be one of your problems. But remember this important fact because it could be just one of literally hundreds of things that could be happening to you and me. What needs to be emphasized is how important and complex it is to look for these problems. I want you to understand that it is very important to look for biochemical changes and malfunctions. We must approach this enigma from every possible direction and not say. . . ."Well, you've got arthritis and that's it. . . .learn to live with it!"

Something controls joint fluid thickness. Something makes it get thin and that something very frequently is an enzyme called hyaluronidase. If hyaluronidase becomes active, it can do many things; one of which is to make the joint fluid thinner.

What makes hyaluronidase active? What stops it? Where does it come from? Why does aspirin help arthritics? Does aspirin have something to do with hyaluronidase activity? Do you have any idea what the most important single chemical is that stimulates hyaluronidase to liquefy the joint fluid? It is. . . .

LEAD

Lead poisoning is something that each and every one of us has in our bodies right now. But lead is not the only culprit.

How much magnesium does it take to shut off hyaluronidase activity?

Why are Vitamin A levels usually low in arthritics?

How can deoxycorticosterone, an adrenal gland hormone

which aggravates arthritis, be changed into cortisone, which helps arthritics, by the use of Vitamin C?

What about bioflavinoids and hesperidin? Are they helpful in hyaluronidase suppression?

What does magnesium have to do with it and how much do you have in your body?

These kinds of questions could go on and on and yet we are still dealing with just one of the many aspects of the arthritis problem. If a proper and adequate study is made of the individual and as many of these aspects tested and treated as possible, there can be no doubt, no question but that arthritis can be altered.

I believe that you are beginning to see how immense this problem really is; not how to live with it, but how to get rid of it.

By the time you finish with this book, you will be aware of a treatment program that has the largest percentage of cure or effectiveness anywhere in the world.

By reducing arthritis to its component parts, we can outline a therapeutic program to correct the components. Here is the breakdown of just what the enemy called ARTHRITIS is all about.

Arthritis is made up of the following components:
    Virus infection
    Anoxia (absence of oxygen)
    Hypoxia (reduced oxygen)
    Change in cellular permeability
        (cell membranes begin to leak)
    Inflammation Toxicity
    Nutritional deficiency
    Calcium deposits
    Reduced viscosity of the joint fluids
        (the joint fluid gets thinner)
    Reduced lymphatic drainage
    Trophic nerve degeneration
    Lead poisoning
    Mercury poisoning
    Arsenic poisoning
    Mitochondrial inactivity
    Toxic allergic reactions
    Hormonal insufficiency
    Circulatory changes

The above listed are problems, not only of arthritics, but of every degenerative disorder. Each one of these malfunctions has a very effective therapy with which it can be neutralized. When a successful therapy for each single item is used, the result will be very interesting and gratifying. If all twenty of the treatments are performed simultaneously, imagine what the results could be like.

A HORMONE THERAPY FOR ARTHRITIS

One of the therapies that is useful in arthritis is a special kind of hormone treatment. Here is an interesting story of how I came into contact with a genius who took a well-known principle that did not work and, with a very slight change, created a treatment that is outstanding. As long as he used the medicines in a way that would not work, he was supported and cheered by his medical colleagues and the provincial arthritis societies. However, when he used the same medications in a slightly different way, he cured the patients. It was then that he was attacked by the medical establishment and eventually died under unusual circumstances.

INTRODUCTION TO HORMONE THERAPY

(A personal true story from the files of Dr. Alsleben.)

A man came to see me some years ago. He was deformed, crippled and essentially disabled. His efforts and good performance gave him an executive position in a major company. He was scheduled for a series of operations on his knees to enable them to move from their stiffly bent positions. This would not cure or even treat his arthritis. . . .just relieve some pain and hopefully, but only possibly, provide greater mobility with a modicum of comfort. For some relief, comfort and greater mobility, he decided instead to come to me to receive the Ion Extractor Therapy and electronic stimulation.

I work diligently with the man for over a year. His state of health markedly improved. His pain diminished and he was happy and grateful. I, however, was frustrated.

The biggest weapons that I had at the time, nearly twenty years ago, gave him a 30-40% improvement. My weapons were used by perhaps ten physicians in the country at that time. They were good. They achieved a 30-40% improvement in an untreatable case. But that wasn't enough. Then on one of his regular visits, he gave me a pamphlet which he had obtained from Aunt Hazel's Vitamin Village Health Food Store. The pamphlet was about the doctor and his treatment for arthritis. George asked me what I thought about the therapy described in the pamphlet. I was intrigued and eagerly leafed through the booklet.

My friend was shocked and pleased at my apparent open-mindedness. When I had finished studying the pamphlet, I said to him, "There's no explanation of the therapy, but the rationale of hormonal balance is excellent. He states that he has helped more than 15,000 patients. If I were you, George, I'd take a short vacation and go on up and see what it's all about. Let me know what is done for you because if it works, I'd like to use it on my patients."

George was content and his confidence in me as a doctor went up another notch simply because I had his best interest at heart. Two months later, he strolled into the office using a cane instead of crutches and with a smile on his face instead of the resignation to pain and agony.

I couldn't wait to go up to him and ask, "My God, George, what happened to you?"

He laughed and replied, "Well, I sure am glad that you

agreed with my going up to see that doctor because that treatment is literally fantastic. And, it's just hormones in a liquid. All of the pain in my knees is gone and they're loosening up. It's just too hard to believe."

I asked him for the address of the doctor so that I might contact him to find out what he was doing.

"That won't help any," George replied, "the doctor was killed just a while ago."

A secret remedy developed through courage and the privilege of research. An answer to arthritis ignored and suppressed by whatever the powers to be might be. Gone forever, or was it?

I went to the doctor's home and spoke with the family. I gathered a healthy respect for the kind of resistance that the doctor received from his colleagues and the enormous efforts that were made to shut him up or to close him down. His final tragic death seemed to be the result of foul play.

The therapeutic concept was to deliver the various kinds of hormones that reduce inflammation and promote protein build-up in a way that would minimize the side-effects and maximize the benefits.

I used the formula myself and was significantly impressed with the results. In fact, I was overwhelmed. But what was it. . . .and why did it work? More than that, what could be wrong with it? The hormones dissolved in the miracle solution were hormones that are produced in everyone's body, but mixed in a special way.

HORMONE FACTS

The therapeutic effects of some of these hormones should be understood so that you can realize the benefits and the negatives of these substances if you should decide to use them.

Adrenal Hormones

1. Depending on the hormone selected, they enhance or decrease the amount of sodium retained in the body. They are necessary for proper carbohydrate metabolism.

2. The presence of the adrenal gland hormones increases the concentration of potassium in the blood plasma. There will also be an increased breakdown of cells which release more potassium into the plasma.

3. The adrenal hormones increase the amount of sugar stored in the liver and muscles as glycogen. There will be an increase in the absorption of sugar from the intestines with an increase in the amount appearing in the blood.

4. The adrenal hormones can cause an increased breakdown of protein in the body. The protein breakdown products will also appear in the blood.

5. The action of the adrenal hormones increases the fat in the liver.

6. The adrenal hormones inhibit the process of inflammation and reduce the migration of the white blood cells.

7. The adrenal hormones increase the output of hydrochloric acid and pepsin in the stomach and the enzyme tripsinogen from the pancreas.

8. When it is given, it reduces the pituitary output of adrenocorticotrophic hormone (ACTH) which in turn results in a decreased activity of the adrenal gland. This results in the reduced production of male and female hormones and protein buildup.

We can see a number of significant physiological effects occurring from an excess of adrenal hormones, whether produced in the body or taken as a medical therapy.

The giving of adrenal cortical hormone or close family member will cause brief beneficial effects if there is a deficiency or an inflammatory process in operation in the body. But, in a very short while, the decrease of the other adrenal cortical hormones results in an imbalance of the endocrine hormones and a considerable breakdown wasting of the individual.

EFFECTS OF ESTROGEN
FEMALE HORMONES

The female hormones are produced in the body of the female in the ovary and the adrenal gland. In the male, the female hormone is produced in the adrenal gland.

Estrogen, female hormones, does the following:

1. Estrogen can cause an increased incorporation of amino acids into the protein structures of certain tissues.

2. It assists in an improvement of RNA buildup.

3. Estrogen causes an increased oxygen metabolism in certain tissues.

4. Estrogen causes a slight sodium retention.

5. Estrogen can assist in an increased deposit of calcium in the bone.

6. The presence of an adequate amount of estrogen will lead to a reduction of fat in the liver, and lipoproteins and cholesterol in the blood.

Did you know that the estrogens are called female hormones simply because they are present in higher concentrations in females than in males? This is primarily due to the additional estrogen production that occurs in the female ovary at the time of egg production. This means that ladies who are past the egg production age are going to have a deficiency of the female hormone with all of the good things that it can do.

EFFECTS OF TESTOSTERONE
MALE HORMONES

Testosterone is called the male hormone because it is in

higher concentrations in the male because it is produced in the testicle as well as the adrenal gland.

One of the common functions of these hormones is to assist in calcium retention in the bones and in protein buildup in the cells. Women who are in the menopausal age usually, sometime after the age of 45, will have a gradual loss of effects from calcium supplementation unless a hormone stimulant is given.

TRADITIONAL TREATMENTS FOR ARTHRITIS

Today, physicians throughout the United States will treat arthritis with four things: pain relievers, anti-inflammatory drugs, some form of cortisone, and a pat on the back.

Here is the sequence of events if the traditional therapies are used:

1. A temporary and short-lived improvement in the general condition. A reduced inflammation.

2. A progressive reduction of male and female hormone production with a resulting calcium depletion and protein wasting.

3. The progressive symptoms of cortisone side-effects are due to a relative excess of cortisone causing other hormones to decrease.

The physician will usually stop the therapy before too

long because the complications begin to become worse than the disease. The primary reason for why the hormonal therapy was good for my friend was because all of the hormones were used together and in balance. Something else that made the therapy unique. It was its unusual method of administration. The hormones were administered under the tongue with the concept that some of the absorption would be through the lymphatic system allowing more of it to come in direct contact with the problem area.

Since we have been working with the preparation, we have developed ways of increasing its lymphatic absorption. The main advantage in this approach is the fact that the hormones will have a longer useful life if they can be kept away from the liver for a while. If the absorption is directly into the blood stream, the liver will rapidly destroy the hormones.

The result of this type of administration was an increased positive hormones effect without as much negative side-effect. Some of the processes by which the hormones are broken down are called conjugation or deconjugation. If the adrenal hormone cortisone were to be injected intravenously, one-half of the total material would be out of the body in four hours. Within two days, 93% of the hormone will have passed out of the body; the major portion of it via the urine with lesser portions through the stool and the skin.

Detoxification of hormones takes place with the aid of a detoxifier called glucuronic acid. If the liver is not working properly, this detoxification will not occur. Consequently, there will be an inadequate breakdown of the cortisone which will then result in retention of sodium and the swelling that comes as a side-effect of cortisone administration.

Are you beginning to see how you can help yourself mentally and nutritionally?

We could find out what the detoxifier glucuronic acid is made from and either take the glucuronate itself or take the components of which it is made as a nutritional supplement.

Obviously the liver will work much more efficiently if it has had the benefits of general body detoxification and cleansing. If a nutritional and herbal approach could be used to reduce the total level of toxic materials in the body, the liver would have a greater capacity to concentrate its wonder-working powers on other functions.

Also, if you could increase the blood circulation to the liver and the bile drainage from the liver, its overall functional capability must improve.

A similar type of detoxification principal is experienced by the male hormone testosterone and the female hormone estrogen. Because the male hormone tends to survive for a longer time in the body, we would tend to see a masculinization of a woman who is no longer producing an adequate amount of female hormone to balance the male hormone; thus the importance of a balanced formula.

At this point, it will be important to review what cortisone does to you. Please realize that you are producing cortisone in your body all the time, but when you take it in medicinal form, you will exaggerate its functions. Here is what cortisone does for you:

THE EFFECTS OF CORTISONE

Elevates blood sugar
Reduces carbohydrate oxidation
Increases glycogen buildup
Decreases conversion of carbohydrate to fat
Increases breakdown of protein to fat
Decreases protein buildup
Reduces the protein structure of the bone
Increases fat breakdown
Increases the transfer of fat from the tissues to the liver
Causes a greater excretion of waste through the urine
Reduces the action and the amount of thymic and lymphatic tissue
Causes a reduction of the white blood cells called the lymphocytes
Increases the large white blood cells
Increases the red blood cells
Increases the secretion of hydrochloric acid and pepsinogen in the stomach. This is what can lead to an increased ulcer formation risk.
Increases the breakdown of muscle tissue
Impairs the cellular use of sulfur and amino acids

It must be remembered that anything that can impair the functions of the liver will decrease the body's ability to get rid of the secreted adrenal hormones. This is the primary problem in cortisone therapy; how to give enough cortisone, or one of its derivatives, so that there will be an effect and yet not too much so that the side-effects do not occur.

And now to summarize the female hormone story once again. What are the most important functions of the female hormones?

ACTIONS OF THE FEMALE HORMONE ESTROGEN

Increases the buildup of proteins in the tissues and bones
Increases the calcium retention in the bones
Increases the movement of hydrogen within the enzyme systems to increase available energy.

ACTIONS OF THE MALE HORMONE TESTOSTERONE

Increased rate of metabolism
Increased rate of red blood cell formation
Increased extracellular fluid volume
Increased sex urge, both male and female

The excess use of powerful adrenal hormones such as cortisone and its derivatives in the treatment of arthritis is inexcusable. This is especially true if the hormone is of the cortisone type. There will be a feedback loop to the pituitary gland to stop producing the hormone that stimulates the adrenal cortex gland. This will result in the reduction of the manufacture of all 60 of its hormones. There will be an increased loss of calcium and increased potential of ulcer formation and the eventual depletion of hydrochloric acid substances from the stomach.

Ultimately, cortisone administration will be a disaster. For a short while, patients may feel relieved, but in the long run, they will be much closer to self-destruction. Unless the adrenals are stimulated at the same time that they are depressed, and unless the proper nutrients are supplied which will reconstitute the hormone production, and unless other measures are taken to protect the body's cells from an excessive loss of nutrients, the entire biochemistry and physiology of the body will be disturbed.

Now you can see why the use of any form of hormone therapy must be carefully and scientifically compounded and administered.

TO GET BACK TO ARTHRITIS

Let's look up the word ARTHRITIS in the medical books and see just what kinds of ingredients it really has. What does the person with arthritis actually have?

PHYSICAL ASPECTS: The arthritic person has:

stiffness	deformity (sometimes)
pain	joint discomfort
lack of mobility	inflammation

CHEMICAL ASPECTS: The arthritic person has:

decreased adrenal gland function
changes in the calcium/phosphorus ratio
lead poisoning which activates the enzyme hyaluronidase
which liquifies joint fluid reducing joint lubrication and
increasing joint friction
increased blood potassium
decreased cellular potassium
changes in the blood acid level
reduced hydrochloric acid production

PHYSIOLOGIC ASPECTS: The arthritic person has:

reduced circulation
nutritional deficiencies
allergic reactions
toxic reactions
neurological disturbances or imbalances
psychologic trauma
neurologic trauma

CONSTRUCTING A BATTLE PLAN

The next thing that we can do is to list these things in a
working battle plan.

Let us try to imagine all the things that could have happened in your body which could eventually result in what certain people would call "arthritis."

1. You could have an hereditary problem.
2. You could have a poisoning from a heavy metal, a gas, a detergent or an industrial chemical.
3. You could have a hormone imbalance.
4. You could have a nerve trauma or imbalance.
5. You could have an injury.
6. You could have a chemical enzyme malfunction.

At this point, we are already ahead of most of the people in the medical world because we now have a basis upon which to attack the problem. If you look at the list, you will see that the only item that is not readily treatable is the item of heredity. Everything else is treatable. Contemplate for a moment what would happen if an arthritic were to get an effective therapy for each of the treatable component parts?

The answer is - the condition will be improved, perhaps markedly so.

As you consider these shocking words, bear one fact in mind. By the time the individual is so contorted, twisted and bent that he or she is unable to dress themselves, we would obviously have expended an enormous span of time. We would have a difficult task identifying the time when the disease first started. When does a disease start?

Try these questions, they might be easier. When does a

dam become unsafe? Is it when the water pours through a hole in its side? Or is it when the first crack appears? You could even take this kind of logic out to its final degree. Did the problem with the dam begin when the very first design was conceived?

If you think of the worst case of arthritis you have ever seen, you must now realize it differs from the slightest case only as a matter of degree. Could such a devastating end result be caused by poison, a trauma, a virus, a bacteria, an allergy, a hormone imbalance, an abnormal nerve transmission and so on?

Could it be caused by any one of them? If it is possible that a single component is going to be the cause. . . .what would it most likely be?

What single cause would have sufficient destructive power to render some normal people totally destroyed in a matter of years and yet others totally unscathed?

A MOST LIKELY CAUSE OF DISEASE

There is only one thing that could fulfill that criteria. . . INFECTION. Assume that infection is really the answer. Is it possible that infection as a single component would render an individual an invalid? Could it do that all by itself? The thought should be hitting you just about now. Of course not. It is not just one of the causes all by itself. It is all of them. . . .interrelated and at the same time. But there is no doubt that infection can be a major factor.

ARTHRITIS MICROBE DISCOVERED

In 1895, a physician delving deeply into the phenomenon of arthritis made a remarkable discovery. He made the assumption that a micro-organism was the culprit in the case of arthritis. Perhaps it was not unusual that Dr. Schuller was looking for microbes. Microbe hunting was a pursuit in vogue in his time. Pasteur, Koch, Jenner and dozens of courageous physicians were looking for relief for suffering for money or perhaps fame. The "microbe" had just been discovered and Schuller set about to find one of his own.

He consistently cultured one micro-organism from the synovial joint fluids of his patients with arthritis. He was also able to demonstrate the same microbe in the tissues of the joint. His work was presented repeatedly before the forum of the most elite organization of his specialty. He published his findings several times in journals having an international circulation and yet they fell into oblivion for the next sixty years. . .even in his own country, Germany. When other experts in the same field were writing historical chronologies of research in the field of arthritis, they would strangely leave Schuller's name and work out.

BACTERIAL CAUSE OF ARTHRITIS CONFIRMED

The only extensive re-evaluation of Schuller's work was done at John's Hopkins University in the year 1905. Dr. Fayerweather duplicated Dr. Schuller's microbe hunt and came to the same conclusion. . .exactly. However, his work also fell into oblivion. His name was not to be mentioned in the followup surveys. The cause for rheumatoid arthritis was uncovered twice and twice it was ignored and lost.

It is inconceivable that Schuller's micro-organism has been missed by competent investigators all over the world. Only extensive research probes can find some mention of it by Rosenow, Margolis, Dorsey, Stein and Benedek.

During the convention of the DEUTSCHE GRESELL-SHAFT FUR SHIRURGIE, Schuller gave a paper on the bacteria that causes arthritis. Listen to this quotation:

"In the fresh preparations individual cocci, or more commonly, short bacilli, either singly or in short chains and containing two shining polar spore bodies could consistently be demonstrated by staining synovial membranes with various aniline dyes. These were seen within the superficial layers, in the deeper foci of inflammation, and occasionally perivascularly."

There it is! A discovery of such monumental importance that it could have saved millions of people from a lifetime of suffering. At first, one has the impulse to laugh at the irony of this tragedy. Then, as you continue to think about it, your heart bleeds with emotions until you simply cannot contain it any longer. Millions of people are sick and dying, all because of the ignorance and stupidity of handfuls of professionals.

Here is the first report about the discovery that was published in the year 1893.

"I here want to make the following brief remarks concerning the morphological and biological characteristics of the bacilli. The bacilli discovered by me resemble short plump rods with a central shallow constriction and with bright or dark polar bodies. As one can observe in well-stained preparations, the polar bodies are round, oval or cylindrical, sitting either close to each other or separated by a minimal bright zone. They do not seem to be spores, but rather condensed protoplasm having peculiar characteristics and taking dyes exceptionally strongly. The spores seem to be formed at the ends or laterally in these portions of the protoplasm. The bacilli are 2 microns long, 1 micron in diameter, and not always straight. They may be flexed at the level of the constriction. I have prepared numerous cultures from the bacilli found by me, not only with those taken from diseased joints, but also those which were inoculated from diseased organs."

Did you hear that?

WHAT IS THE CAUSE OF MANY DISEASES?

KLEPTIC MICROBES

The same organism that causes arthritis can be found in other tissues. Does it do anything in the other organs or tissues? Or would we give its effect another name? What we would call it if it produced a disease of the liver? Would we call it arthritis of the liver? I have never heard of that and neither have you. It would probably be called cirrhosis or hepatitis or even cancer.

Are the pathologies of the body all essentially the same, just changing their names to match locations and a few individual characteristics?

Schuller reported that if he took the bacillus out of a human and put it into a rabbit, the rabbit would develop arthritis. Schuller was not able to determine how the bacillus got into the body in the first place. This was to be discovered thirty years later.

Listen to this statement by Dr. Max Schuller.

"In the inflammatory hyperplastic tissue of the synovial joint capsule and the villi of the capsule, I found cocci and bacilli years ago. This caused me to undertake, by means of a special canula, inoculations from joints not yet opened. The micro-organisms can only be found in the inflamed synovials and villi, not in the joint cavity. I have made 23 punctures in different patients. To my good fortune, I have found the bacilli regularly and at once in the first of these cultures. Depending on the individual cases, many or a few bacilli, at times with cocci, were found. The bacilli could be found in every case. They sit in the usually minute fluid of the joint. The bacilli usually occur within the greatest pathological alteration where massive accumulations of cells and inflammatory proliferation of the prevailing endothelial-like connective tissue cells can be observed. When I

*made cultures from these two different joints of a patient,
either at once or on different occasions, I sometimes
observed only bacilli in these cultures, while at times,
these same cultures seem to be mixed with cocci or
occasionally with diploccci. The cocci uniformly look
similar to the pyogenic cocci found in the tissues of many
other articular conditions due to gonorrhea or
tuberculosis. The pathological process as a whole is, in
my opinion, an independent infectious disease elicited by
the invasion of the bacilli. In man, this rheumatoid
arthritis usually begins with the development of villous
excrescences. The growing villous excrescences always
originate from a determinable part of the synovialis.
they grow more extensively in one direct and therefore
deform the joint capsule. In the shoulder joint, large
excrescences are rarely observed. In the elbow, the
process often begins in the synovialis under the annular
ligament and around the head of the radius. The
anterior and the posterior cavities of the humerus bone
are likewise the seat of this development. In the hand,
the little joint between the ulna and the radius, as well as
the wrist joint, are affected with the disease. The hip
joint is attacked mostly in the very sever cases. Fixation
in extension is produced. The knee joint is very often
affected and can be filled with larger masses of the
villous excrescences. Those behind the lateral ligaments
will give rise to trouble early. Pain on digital pressure is
common."*

THE KILLER WITH A THOUSAND FACES

The cocci-type bacteria that Dr. Schuller described in his punctures and tissue sections, along with the bacilli or occasionally alone, were described by him as being an extreme polymorphism of this organism. Furthermore, he underscored the fact that he observed these cocci to be most frequently present in the atrophic, ankylosing forms of chronic rheumatoid arthritis and that these cocci sometimes occurred as diplocci. He did this with a knowledge that few other physicians had until many decades later. **Without knowing the concept of polymorphism, the concept that a microbe could change its shape and characteristics depending on its environment,** one could easily believe to have an entirely different species of cocci at hand. These organisms show an amazing degree of polymorphism.

Is this the explanation for how this organism could have been missed by the tens of thousands of investigators worldwide? Who could know the answer to that one? I remember a hematologist, a blood specialist, who came to my office to check out my darkfield microscope. He had never looked through one before that visit.

We put a drop of blood on the slide and got it all focused up so that it would show the small coccal bacterial forms in the black background. They were there dancing about by the hundreds. I turned the microscope over to him and when he got himself settled, I asked him, "Do you see the small dancing white spots in the black background?" His answer was, "What white spots?"

33

It was the first time that he had ever looked at the blood through that kind of microscope. Perhaps his eyes just couldn't register something that they had not seen before. I said to him, "Just keep looking and when you see them, let me know." About 10 seconds went by and then he suddenly blurted out, "Now I see them, what are they?"

He quickly left and I never saw him again. My guess is that many investigators do not allow themselves to reveal it or they assume that it is not what they were looking for and could be discarded.

Maybe the organism was too difficult for most people to see. Maybe it was too difficult to grow. On the other hand, how could they have missed several textbooks written about it during the last 80 years?

ARTHRITIS MICROBE FOUND AGAIN

Four years after Dr. Schuller's first publication in 1892, a group of investigators repeated Dr. Schuller's work. They were Drs. Bannatyne, Wohlmann and Blaxall. Their work was not as good as Schuller's, but they did do something very interesting. They produced the first culture of this organism from human blood and joint fluid.

Gilbert Bannatyne, a British internist, confirmed in 1896 Schuller's discovery of the presence of the bacilli in synovial and joint connective tissues. He was the first to be successful in culturing the organism from the blood. His textbook was published three times in 1896 and

1904. Hear these words from his books:

"In the microscopic preparations, we found organisms in 24 cases out of 25 rheumatic joints examined. It was a microbe, and it was always the same microbe as far as size and shape, appearance, staining properties and cultural behavior. Sometimes they were present in enormous numbers. Having gained a foothold in the circulation, the microbes pass freely to all organs of the body, thus explaining the symmetry of the disorder and why one joint after another should be involved. The microbes grow and propagate in the synovial membranes, ligaments, bone marrow and cartilaginous structures."

How is it possible that these kinds of verifiable observations were made and published over 80 years ago and yet your family doctor, the arthritis specialist, or the institutional researchers are aware of it?

How can research of this magnitude have been known for more than three-quarters of a century and yet when the specialist is asked why he cannot effectively treat the problem, he shrugs his shoulders and confesses that the cause is not known? How can associations collect and spend hundreds of millions and perhaps billions of dollars over a period of decades and not make a breakthrough in the management of a simple little organism whose very existence is denied?

From the pen of Dr. Blaxall in 1896 comes these words that shed some light on the problems observing these microbes.

"Dr. Bannatyne arrived at the conclusion, from clinical aspects of cases suffering from rheumatoid arthritis, that the disease was due to a micro-organism. And further, that in the microscopic examinations of the synovial fluids from affected joints, they found an organism constant and distinct. They claimed that the organism was specific for arthritis."

At that time, Dr. Blaxall was with the laboratories of the British Institute of Preventive Medicine. He goes on to say more:

"Bannatyne sent the synovial fluid to me for examination. My first attempts to stain the organism in the synovia and to obtain cultures from it resulted in failure. The technique of staining seemed to be the problem. Finally, using aniline methylene blue, I saw it. Microscopic examinations of the specimens revealed an organism possessing peculiar characteristics. At first sight, it appears to be a diploccocus, the two cocci being distinctly stained, but separated by a clear unstained interval about equal in length to the diameter of either stained end. It turned out that this is a bacillus which exhibits very marked polar staining. I have now stained and examined the synovial fluid from various joints from 18 cases affected with rheumatoid arthritis and, in every one, I have observed the organism which I have just described. But, in the fluids from distended joints due to other causes, I have failed entirely to find them."

THE ORGANISM THAT CRIPPLED THE WORLD

What an incredibly exciting discovery for a handful of physicians to make. What a remarkable achievement to be involved in during one's lifetime. But there is one peculiar aspect of his work and the work of others. They say that they could not see them without a particular type of stain. What kind of microscope were they using? Then they say that they finally discovered a chemical that could stain them and there they were. What about other bacteria present that do not accept a particular stain? Are they to be dismissed?

Dr. Blaxall makes some other comments about the difficulty growing the organisms.

"Cultivation, both anaerobic and aerobic, yielded no apparent results. This might have been due to the small size of the colony or its almost invisible character. Three days in beef broth and it remained perfectly clear, pointing strongly to the conclusion that the synovial fluid contained no ordinary organism. It can be readily understood from the delicate nature of the cultures and the imperfections of the staining methods, that a too great reliance on stained specimens was not advisable. I have also grown the organism in milk, where it appears to flourish, but without causing curdling or precipitation of the casein."

The next few sentences from Blaxall's work are absolutely astonishing.

"As far as I am aware, only one organism has been previously associated with rheumatoid arthritis. This was the organism described by Dr. Schuller. After comparing my findings with his, it is obvious that the organism described by Schuller differs markedly from the one under discussion. In fact, the only points of resemblance are the polar staining and the easy discoloration. It appears to me to be indisputable that the organism of Schuller is not that which was discovered by Bannatyne."

Well, as you can see, the mystery deepens. Are we to believe now that there are more than one type of organism that could cause arthritis in a joint? Could there be many? As armchair bacteriologists are we, or are you, going to demonstrate that you are smarter than the best scientists and the hundreds of millions of dollars given to foundations and societies perpetually promising a cure around the corner? Which corner are they talking about? What is going to be the conclusion that you will arrive at which should win you the Nobel Price. . . whatever that is. Let me help you. Could it be that one kind of bacteria has the ability to change into many kinds?

In 1896, Dr. Bannatyne wrote these words:

"From the discovery made by Dr. Woklmaun and myself, no doubt remains in my mind that rheumatoid arthritis is caused by micro-organisms which we have found to exist in the joint fluids and tissues. The presence of these organisms gives rise to acute inflammatory changes

leading to ulcerations, erosion and destruction of the hard, as well as the soft, tissues. The questions is - how do the organisms gain access to the joint spaces in the first place? The probability is that they set up an endarteritis in one of the small vessels on the surface of the synovial membrane, with a diffuse cell exudation, and this by extension and rupture, liberates them for further mischief. Under the microscope, the synovial membrane is seen to be infiltrated with newly-formed connective tissue cells. The blood vessels are dilated and their walls are thickened. Here and there are small collections of leukocytes surrounding them. The microbes seem to collect wherever there are round cells."

Dr. Schuller's discovery could have shortened or ended human misery related to that disorder. His discovery failed to receive any understanding from his colleagues. One could even question if they made up the differences just to deny him the credit for whipping one of the worst diseases known to man. Despite his publications, presentations and demonstrations of the microbes, despite the fact that his work was substantiated and confirmed by Bannatyne, the work was quickly forgotten. Fortunately, their names were occasionally quoted so that they at least survived to this day to enable this article to be written. Even the name of Fayerweather, a third man of this period, was totally forgotten, despite his brilliant observations.

In 1905, Fayerweather was a clinical assistant in orthopedic surgery at John's Hopkins Hospital. It was while he was working in the laboratories of Tufts College

Medical School in Boston that he published his information confirming Schuller's discovery.

Fayerweather repeated Schuller's techniques on patients with rheumatoid arthritis. He found the bacilli exactly where Schuller said they would be. He found them in the lymphatic channels where the white blood cells aggregate in the largest numbers. How could these bacteria continue to be there and not be devoured by the white blood cells? It's an interesting question, isn't it?

Fayerweather made this conclusion - there was no difference between acute articular rheumatic arthritis and infectious polyarthritis chronic villosa. He concludes one of his documents with this observation:

"It is surprising that with the great interest in bacteriological research in this country, we should have failed to recognize the significance of Schuller's and Bannatyne's work. . .no satisfactory work has been done in the bacteriological research of their cases."

We personally performed a research of the literature of bacteriology and rheumatology in America since 1905. The indepth probe failed to produce any articles on the bacteria that was discovered by Fayerweather, other than the articles that he himself wrote while at John's Hopkins.

A patient once asked me, "Could it be that most of the medical profession around the world does not want to know how to correct arthritis?"

As every physician goes through his or her training, they will come across a few cases where arthritis was created in a patient by the administration of penicillin, sulfur drugs or certain viruses. In 1949, the American Rheumatism Association prepared a survey summary of what could be done about rheumatoid arthritis. More than a half-century had gone by since the discovery of the infective nature of the disease. The disease had become so widespread and catastrophic as a public health disaster that associations sprung up to associate with it. Here is a list of what the largest association for arthritis in the world determined that the medical community of this country was able to do for victims of the disease. The list is impressive, as I am sure you will agree.

Rest
Hygiene
Nutrition
Salicylate drugs
Physical therapy
Occupational therapy
Psychotherapy
Rehabilitation
Transfusions
X-ray
Climate control
Cortisone
ACTH pituitary hormone

That is what they recommended. Did it work?

Here is a list of treatments that they considered to be absolutely useless.

> Vaccine therapy
> Foreign protein therapy
> Vitamins
> Specific drugs
> Glandular preparations
> Dietary fads
> Fever therapy

That is what they said would not work. But as we now know, the therapies they said couldn't work, did work. The paradox is frightening. As a result of this attitude, the arthritic patient has nothing to look forward to except misery. And so it goes again. . .tens of millions, perhaps hundreds of millions, share the fate of misery.

The offices of arthritis doctors are filled to the brim with cripples who stay crippled. And this is in spite of the fact that there are at least five therapeutic procedures that can practically eliminate the problem. The evidence has been generated by medical investigators, but when it is given to some sort of medical authority, it is ignored and very uncomfortable retaliatory forces are brought to bear upon the researchers or therapists.

If one carefully evaluates some of the therapies of traditional medicine which supposedly help, one finds a common denominator known as **"the old time medicine."**

There is an interference with the bacterial allergic inflammatory reaction cycle between the bacteria and the injured cell. Most of the time, the interference is a temporary one. The treatment is followed by relief, which is followed by a more severe return of the disease. One of the therapies that has been advocated by the arthritic establishment is called Gold Therapy. Many arthritic patients are familiar with it and it is still being used today. In high doses, Gold Therapy is effective. However, in high doses, it is damaging, destructive and sometimes fatal. To avoid these objectionable side-effects, the dosage of Gold Therapy has become very much reduced in order to make it safe. However, at the lower and safe doses, it is useless.

The same can be said for ACTH and cortisone. High doses work and destroy, while the lower, safer doses are ineffective. In each case when the therapy is stopped, the arthritis almost always returns. . .worse than it was before the therapy.

The authoritative representatives of arthritis have said that vaccine therapy does not work. How absurd! Vaccines are the most specific treatments that one could ever hope to have. To blatantly and across the board say that vaccine therapy does not work, if it is a true statement, simply means that the correct vaccine is not being used. To say that vaccine therapy does not work seems to be an obvious attempt to deprive you of receiving it.

According to medical literature, research papers,

experimental studies, clinical trials and major textbooks that I have found in the largest medical libraries in the world, the use of a specific vaccine would probably reduce or eliminate the disease.

You find that hard to believe? Listen to this:

ANOTHER MAGIC BULLET!

Twenty-four cases of rheumatoid arthritis, ranging in age from 20 to 66, having had arthritis from between 2 months to 20 years were given a specific vaccine for the bacteria that is involved in the production of the disease. Here are the results:

One of the 24 had a mild degree of improvement.
Twenty of the 24 were totally corrected.

What kinds of cases are these? Here is a typical example:

A 55 year old housewife with progressive rheumatoid arthritis for 17 years. The condition progressively involved more and more of the peripheral joints and she became increasingly incapacitated. The patient had never had any major medical or surgical disease until three years before her hysterectomy, followed in one year by pneumonia. The first symptoms of arthritis were painful and swollen wrists with limitation of motion. Subsequently the ankles, elbows and knees became involved. Later both shoulders and the fingers became involved with the same pathological process. She took high doses of aspirin for the severe pain, but was never under proper medical care. She treated herself with patent medicines, all to no avail. Seventeen years later, even the sternoclavicular and breast bone joints were involved. This restricted her breathing. Both shoulders were frozen.

A SPECIFIC VACCINE

A specific vaccine was made from the organism cultured from the tissue and a small injection was given every week. In five weeks, the sternoclavicular and costosternal joints no longer showed swelling. There was no pain. Her breathing was normal. She could walk six blocks for the first time in two years because her knees were better. She gradually improved. By the 14th week, there was no pain or swelling in any joint. She went on to a complete recovery.

HOW DOES A VACCINE IMPROVE IMMUNITY?

How is immunity produced or increased by the injection of a bacterial vaccine? An antigen must come into parenteral contact with the tissue cells in order to cause these cells to develop immunologic capabilities. In the increase in the capability to anchor and destroy the bacterial cells and their constituents, lies the immunizing value of a vaccine. In what tissue should a vaccine be injected? When a vaccine is injected into the blood stream, the bacterial cells might be taken up largely by the fixed and mobile phagocytes. Then antigenic constituents liberated from the bacterial cells will ultimately be carried by the circulation to all parts of the body. An outstanding difference between the injection of a vaccine into the blood stream and into some tissue, particularly the skin, would seem to be that in the blood stream, vaccine is rapidly taken up by the phagocytes, while in the tissues, it comes into more prolonged contact with the cutaneous tissue.

Much knowledge has been gained recently with regard to the structural nature of bacterial vaccines. Generally, the S or smooth form of the microbes is pathogenic while the R or rough form is not. Correspondingly, a vaccine made of the S form is believed to possess the property of calling forth defensive mechanisms on the part of the host, while a vaccine made from the R form is believe to lack this property. An interesting finding is that when virulent S forms are grown in mediums containing some homologous immune serum, they rapidly dissociate into R forms.

VACCINE AGAINST WHAT?
AND THE DISCOVERY AND NAMING OF THE KLEPTIC MICROBE

We have spent considerable space detailing the work of some of great scientists who have gone before us who observed a microbe in arthritic joints. We have also observed this same microbe and are convinced it is in fact a pleomorphic organism, which is associated with many chronic disorders including, very specifically, arthritis. It was named by us the "Kleptic" microbe because we do not see it as a voracious destroyer of tissue, but instead see it as a robber of energy from the defenders of health, the components of the immune system.

Active, virile immune cells are observed under the microscope to become sluggish and almost lifeless after contact with these high-energy microbes. (For a more detailed explanation, see THE KLEPTIC MICROBE by Alsleben and Donsbach.)

More important, we have been able to either significantly reduce or completely eliminate this form of microbial contamination from the blood by a very special infusion. Within 2 hours after the beginning of the infusion, a blood sample that was formerly teeming with these tiny microbes is without evidence of their presence. In addition, we cultured the microbe and are now using an immune modulating blueprint which can be self-administered to prevent its recurrence.

This procedure may truly signal the end of suffering for countless millions of arthritics. By a wholistic cleansing of the body as a whole, by removing the energy thief who reduces our ability to defend ourselves and by stimulating body defenses by an appropriate *immune modulating blueprint*™, the spector of arthritis could vanish.

NUTRITIONAL ASPECTS OF ARTHRITIS

The use of hormone balancing and the destruction of the Kleptic Microbe are only two of the approaches that must be utilized in the proper treatment of the arthritic complex. Any time a wasting disease such as this strikes a person, extensive repair must take place in order to restore normal or near-normal function. You will remember that there are many tissues and many causes involved in the distortion of function called arthritis.

Let us examine some of the nutritional components that should be addressed in this disease.

Over 20 years ago, Drs. E.C. Barton-Wright and W.A. Elliot, physicians at the Rheumatic Clinic in London, England, found that the symptoms of *both* osteo and rheumatoid arthritis were relieved by the use of oral pantothenic acid, one of the B Complex vitamins. According to Baron-Wright, arthritis is caused, at least in part, by insufficient intake of pantothenic acid due to the excessive intake of highly processed foods so common in the Western World.

DR. JOHN M. ELLIS

Dr. John M. Ellis, Chief of Medical Staff at Titus County Memorial Hospital, Mt. Pleasant, TX, has studied another of the B vitamins since 1961. His work on Vitamin B_6 (Pyridoxine) is thoroughly and completely reported in two books which he has written, *"The Doctor Who Looked At Hands"* and *"Vitamin B-6. The Doctor's Report."* His conclusions regarding the role of B_6 in arthritis were as follows: reduced pain in the shoulder, hip and knee areas and a cessation of night-time muscle cramps. The amount of Vitamin B_6 used varied, but the average dose was from 500 to 1,000 mg daily.

DR. ROGER J. WILLIAMS

Dr. Roger J. Williams, the distinguished biochemist who is perhaps responsible for more original work in the field of vitamin research than any living chemist, points out the relationship of Vitamin C, Vitamin A, Vitamin B$_2$ (riboflavin), the minerals calcium and magnesium to arthritis, since it is a "Collagen Disease." Collagen is the elastic protein substance which makes up cartilage which is the cushion material around the joints of the body. Cartilage is subjected to a lot of abuse just from normal motion of the body and requires continual rebuilding to do its job of absorbing the jolts and strains that would destroy bone surfaces if they were not protected by cartilage. The above nutrients play an important part in the normal formation of replacement collagen, which makes up a great portion of cartilage. Therefore, a lack of any one or a deficiency of all of them would impede cartilage cell repair and open the door to arthritic symptoms. We really should bring the drug, cortisone, into discussion since the relief which some obtain from its administration is almost miraculous, but temporary and loaded with side-effects. Just what does cortisone do? The adrenal glands are one of the most important glands we have in the body when we are dealing with stress - and arthritis is certainly a stress disease. The adrenals produce many hormones which are needed to "trigger" functions in the body. One of those functions is rebuilding and maintaining healthy cartilage and connective tissue. Interestingly enough, pantothenic acid, Vitamin C and the mineral potassium are all involved in the normal production of these adrenal hormones, including cortisone. We stress that other hormones produced by the adrenal glands are needed to work in harmony with cortisone for normal functioning. Thus, the use of cortisone alone produces a hormonal imbalance with all kinds of side-effects. One the other hand, the restoring of the above-mentioned nutrients to the dietary intake of an individual will enhance the normal production of all the adrenal hormones. So an absence of any of these vital nutrients could cause poor cartilage repair which, in turn, would lead to arthritis.

The use of "folk remedies" should also be brought into this discussion. Through trial and error, often by accident and without knowing the chemistry behind the effect, some of the most dramatic advances in medicine have been made by lay persons. A favorite remedy for years has been equal parts of cream of tartar and epsom salts in a glass of water morning and night. When we look at the components of these two common ingredients, we can see why there was a certain degree of success in their use. Cream of Tartar is made up largely of potassium and Epsom Salts is primarily magnesium. Both of these minerals have been discussed previously in their relationship to the health of the adrenal glands and the utilization of calcium.

One of the most difficult "folk remedies" to determine its effectiveness is "Certo," a product used by homemakers in the preparation of jams and jellies. It is composed primarily of fruit pectin and until we learned that many arthritics have an extraordinary amount of lead in the blood stream, the answer evaded us. Lead "replaces" calcium in bone structures which leads to all kinds of calcium-related disorders. Pectin renders lead insoluble in the body and so we had the answer. The reason these remedies are sometimes ineffective is that the mechanism by which they work for some may not be the cause of the problems with others. Again, we must emphasize a total approach. Only then can we have some assurance of success in the different types of arthritis.

A TRUE LINK

What this research indicates is that there is a true link between a "chronic degenerative disease" such as arthritis and adequate availability of nutrients. I would like to quote from Dr. Roger J. Williams' book "Nutrition Against Disease."

"Environmental Prevention - While medical education has put a damper on experiments in which the nutrition of arthritics might have been studied and manipulated in an expert fashion, there is excellent reason for thinking that if this were done, sufferers could get real rather than palliative relief. There is even a good possibility that individual arthritics will be able - if they are lucky and make intelligent trials - to hit upon particular nutrients or nutrient combinations which will bring benefit.

I certainly would not want to give the impression that the management of these diseases is simple. But I do affirm the dictum that nutrition should be tried first. On the *basis of reports presently available, the items that certainly need to be considered are niacinamide, pantothenic acid, riboflavin, Vitamin A, Vitamin C, Vitamin B$_6$, magnesium, calcium, phosphorus, and other minerals. The objective is to feed adequately the cells that are involved in keeping the bones, joints and muscles in healthy condition.*

It could not be said more clearly. Only one cautionary word. Do not use fragmented nutritional supplements. Find a formula that contains all the nutrients and use that as your foundation product. If, after you have used it for some time, you find there is an additional need for some nutrient - Vitamin C as an example - add it to your program. Remember that all these substances work as a team and the total effect of all is far greater than individual effects.

Here is an example of what we would consider to be a complete food supplement with emphasis on the nutrients which researchers have found of assistance in arthritis:

Vitamin A	25,000 IU
Vitamin D	400 IU
Vitamin B1	50 mg
Vitamin B2	50 mg
Vitamin B6	100 mg
Vitamin B12	500 mcg
Vitamin C	1,500 mg
Vitamin E	400 mg
Niacinamide	50 mg

Folic Acid	400 mg
Biotin	25 mcg
Pantothenic Acid	1,500 mg
Choline	40 mg
Inositol	50 mg
Para Amino Benzoic Acid	50 mg
Glutamic Acid HCI	100 mg
Bromelain	100 mg
Citrus Pectin	150 mg
Lemon Bioflavinoids	100 mg
Calcium	1,000 mg
Magnesium	400 mg
Iron	15 mg
Iodine	.225 mg
Manganese	25 mg
Potassium	99 mg
Chromium	150 mcg
Zinc	25 mg
Copper	2 mg
Selenium	150 mcg
Adrenal Substances	100 mg

Try this restorative, rejuvenating program and be blessed two times. First when you find that you can control and discipline your body and secondly when the freedom from pain and inconvenience of disease is restored to you. Remember that self-discipline is less limiting than disease.

NIGHTSHADE ALLERGY

Several worthwhile reports have been published on the total restriction of the Nightshade family of foods for those who have arthritis. It appears that certain susceptible individuals cannot tolerate those foods from the Nightshade family of plants (bell pepper, paprika, tomato, white potato, eggplant) and, if they are consumed, arthritic stiffness, pain, inflammation, etc., sets in. The exact mechanism or even the offending ingredient in these plants is not known with certainty, so my advise is rather simple. If the preceding program is not successful for you, try eliminating these foods. They are not an absolute essential in the diet and planning your menu without them should not be difficult task.

NIACINAMIDE

Osteoarthritis may respond to extra amounts of the B vitamin, niacinamide. Dr. William Kaufman, a medical pioneer in the nutritional approach to disease, found that a basic pellagra diet high in niacinamide was very effective in the treatment of this disorder. Although his work only indicated the use of 100-150 mg of supplemental niacinamide daily, we have found that up to 500 mg is often even more effective.

NOTE: Pantothenic acid is probably the equivalent for the rheumatoid arthritic. We normally suggest 1,500 mg of pantothenic acid for what appears to be a severe deficiency in some who suffer from rheumatoid arthritis.

GOUTY ARTHRITIS AND CHERRIES

The pain that is related to gout has variously been described as "exquisite," "horrible," "tortuous," etc. There can be no question that the condition exists when you have it because of the pain and swelling. It not only afflicts the big toe as in the famous "Jiggs" cartoon character, but can afflict the hands, wrist, elbow, etc. The purine-restricted diet, which is recommended for gout, is based upon the gout sufferer's inability to properly metabolize one of the waste products of protein breakdown, uric acid. This uric acid accumulates in the body and tends to crystallize which irritates surrounding structures.

However, research has uncovered some other interesting possibilities. According to biochemist George Brooks and social psychologist Ernst Mueller, "a tendency to gout is a tendency to the executive suite." In the prestigious *"Journal of The American Medical Association"* (02-07-66), it states "Higher than average uric acid content in the serum and high intelligence or intellectual attainment are related."

Possibly the physiologic explanation of this is that the stress associated with "high achievers" may inhibit an enzyme system that is needed in the body to handle such situations. The other interesting aspect is that the possibility exists that a higher than normal level of uric acid may, in some way, stimulate the higher cortical (reasoning) centers in the brain. Then wouldn't all of us want more uric acid? Not necessarily so. Many have rather high levels of uric acid and suffer no problems with gout but a few have severe problems with this disorder as their uric acid levels rise.

Maybe we have an answer. Dr. Ludwig Blau suggested, after many successful cases, that cherries and/or cherry juice have a beneficial effect on gout. His candid "I don't know what cherries or cherry juice contain that helps to alleviate gout, but I know it does," is reminiscent of the many other folklore remedies that work, but the scientific reason has not been justified at this point. The mechanism seems to revolve around keeping the uric acid in solution and not letting it crystallize. But exactly how this is accomplished is not clear.

The amount of cherries that are effective varies, but six or more on a daily basis seems to be a good prevention with considerably more for therapeutic use. Most varieties of cherries seem to work, but the "sour cherry" is the easiest to grow and the most pesticide free. They are not sour when ripe so the name is somewhat misleading.

CARTILAGE EXTRACT

Chondroitin sulfate, a substance which is found in plentiful supply in cartilage of animals and sharks, has the ability to liquefy the synovial fluid which literally lubricates the joints. We have previously discussed that in many cases of arthritis, the synovial fluid has become very thick and non-lubricating in the joint, leading to wear and tear. Many independent research studies have demonstrated that in animals and humans with arthritis, the addition of cartilage extract containing chondroitin sulfate will reduce the symptoms of stiffness, swelling and pain.

It has been so successful that it has been double-blind tested against the non-steroidal, anti-inflammatory drugs and the somewhat popular gold shots and come out as the treatment of choice. Although we start out patients with a hefty amount, once the response cycle has occurred, it is reduced so that the long-term maintenance prescription is relatively small.

SUPEROXYGENATION

The use of hydrogen peroxide and other oxygen-rich substances as a home treatment for arthritis have been the topic of many conversations. Most doctors are immediately negative regarding these liquid oxygen preparations since they believe, erroneously, that the release of the oxygen is in the form of a free radical that will harm the cell. On the other hand, people who suffer from arthritis symptoms and who usually have far less inhibition for using what appears to be a simple remedy, have reported some rather excellent results with this therapy.

One of the authors (Dr. Donsbach) has had considerable experience with the use of all forms of oxygen enhancing therapies. It is his opinion that oxygen is a first line ingredient in any health program and will assist anyone with any type of disease to recover faster. The reason for this opinion is based upon the following two functions of oxygen that are well recognized in the scientific world:

1. Oxygen is one of the key ingredients by which the body manufactures energy. Combining oxygen with glucose creates the chemical ATP, which we recognize as energy. Very rarely is glucose deficient in one's diet, but it is most common to see oxygen deficiency in everyone who is ill with any kind of disease. When energy levels fall, all functions in the body are inhibited because every one of them requires a plentiful supply of energy to complete their work. Think about it for a moment, life is energy - no energy - no life! When an individual is suffering from any kind of malady, the need for oxygen is even more evident because of all the repair and replacement that is going on.

2. Oxygen is extensively used by the body as a detoxifier. Every metabolic function which helps to maintain the status quo in the body is also continually releasing metabolic waste products into the body. These products can be toxic but, by combining them with oxygen, they are rendered quite harmless and are readily removed from the body.

These two very important functions, energy enhancement and detoxification, are the dream of every physician who deals with illness. Relief of pain is not uncommon at all with oxygen increase in the bloodstream and this can be accomplished by the use of drinking oxygen-rich cocktails, infusing oxygen-rich liquids directly into the blood stream and by introducing ozone into the rectum where it converts to hydrogen peroxide and eventually oxygen and is absorbed into the heavy network of veins in that area.

We use all of these methods as well as immersing the body into a whirlpool which has been heavily saturated with hydrogen peroxide, which is 94% oxygen, at Hospital Santa Monica in Mexico and Institut Santa Monica in Poland.

ION EXTRACTOR THERAPY

For many years, alternative physicians have been using a procedure called intravenous chelation therapy for the arthritis problem. As you will remember, lead is often a factor in arthritis. In fact, it is often involved in many of the problems of modern man. Contamination with this toxic metal is widespread and has been cited as a factor in many neuro-muscular diseases, mental problems, etc.

The use of the di-sodium salt of a synthetic amino acid, ethylene-diamine-tetracetic acid (EDTA) has been found to literally wrap itself around lead in the body and carry it with the EDTA as it is eliminated from the body. One of the authors (Dr. Alsleben) was the first physician to carry out extensive chelation procedures in an office out-patient setting. Before that, EDTA infusions were done only in hospitals.

During Dr. Alsleben's thousands of treatments administered in a variety of conditions, he was able to perfect a very special formula which is a great advancement over the ones which have been in use for many years. Not only is there far less strain on the patient and far less possibility of any side-effects, but the results are seen to a greater extent and in far less time. This provides an obvious savings in time and money. Dr. Alsleben calls this "Ion Extractor Therapy" and has registered the formulation and protocol.

In certain patients with the symptoms of arthritis, this treatment is so productive of results that it is almost unbelievable; but it is not always this dramatic. This only points out the variables on the etiology of this condition of the body.

LIVER - KIDNEY - BOWEL CLEANSING FAST

One of the most important factors in any disease condition is the detoxification of the body. It should also follow that such a detoxification can be an excellent means of preventing disease and promoting good health. The following is a simple three day program which accomplishes detoxification of the major organs involved in retaining toxins in the body.

Materials needed:

1. From 12 to 16 lemons daily, depending on size. (If fresh lemons are unavailable, you can buy pure concentrated lemon juice.)

2. From 2 to 3 quarts of distilled water daily.

3. A small amount of honey.

4. One bottle of an herb combination containing garlic, black cohosh, chaparral, fenugreek, red sage and goldenseal.

5. One bottle of dietary fiber. (May be called bran tablets.)

FIRST DAY: One and one-half cups of freshly squeezed (or the equivalent of concentrate) lemon juice, mixed with 2 quarts of distilled water and a little honey for palatability. This will be your total intake of fluid and food for the day, so you may sip on it constantly. Take 2 of the herb tablets both morning and evening. Take 8 dietary fiber tablets in the morning and 8 in the afternoon with a 10 ounce glass of the lemon mixture.

SECOND DAY: Repeat the mixing of approximately 2 1/2 quarts of the lemon juice-distilled water and honey mixture and consume it during the day. Use 3 of the herb tablets morning and evening and 8 dietary fiber tablets twice daily.

THIRD DAY: Repeat the mixing approximately 2 1/2 quarts of of the lemon juice, distilled water and honey mixture and consume it during the day. Use 4 of the herb tablets morning and evening and 8 dietary fiber tablets twice daily.

FOURTH AND FIFTH DAY: Stop using the lemon juice, distilled water and honey mixture, but continue the use of 2 herb tablets morning and evening. Also, use 8 dietary fiber tablets morning and afternoon. Drink all you wish of tomato juice, carrot juice, grape juice (dilute the grape juice with about 1/3 spring water) or other vegetable or fruit juices. Eliminate citrus juices. Consume all the fresh spring water you wish.

SIXTH AND SEVENTH DAY: Add raw fruits and vegetables to your regime, maintaining herb and dietary fiber tablet intake as before. Consume all the fresh juices that you wish.

EIGHTH DAY: Add yogurt and/or cottage cheese. Continue dietary fiber and herb tablets twice daily as before.

NINTH DAY: Add lightly-steamed vegetables to allowable foods. Reduce dietary fiber tablet intake to 12 daily and continue taking 4 herb tablets on a daily basis.

TENTH DAY: If desired, add small portion of meat to one meal - seeds, nuts or eggs are just as acceptable. Reduce dietary fiber tablets to 4 in the morning and 4 in the afternoon and continue taking 4 herb tablets daily.

ELEVENTH DAY AND FORWARD: Follow the Creative Restoration Diet; adjust dietary fiber tablets according to personal need. Lower bowel gas and foul odored stools are indications of increased need for dietary fiber. You may now discontinue the herb tablets.

FASTING

Many who read this book will desire to have the results that are discussed but are a bit squeamish about the three day fast. Questions such as these are often asked:

Q. Can I fast if I also have hypoglycemia?

A. Yes, you can. Hypoglycemia, much the same as diabetes, is triggered by the ingestion of sugar. Since the fast does not contain any sugar, we do not trigger the condition. If you are taking insulin injections, you must check with your doctor as to your participation in a fast.

Q. Can I continue to work while on this program?

A. Yes, you can. Often time, an individual feels stronger on the third day of the fast than they did before the fast.

Q. What signs can I look for to see if the program is working?

A. Some individuals have minor stomach nausea and/or headaches. These are the people who are the most toxic and the body is having some trouble eliminating toxins from the bloodstream rapidly enough. However, the first and most common sign, often at the end of the second or in the third day, is the lessening of pain and stiffness.

Q. Will I get weak?

A. It is very unusual for this to occur. Remember on the fourth day, you are beginning to consume some food again.

Biologically-oriented doctors consider fasting to be the most important curative measure in the treatment of arthritis. Some may disagree as to the length of the fast. I happen to believe that it is far safer, more practical and even more beneficial to limit fasting to 3 days. This can be repeated every 10 days until the desired response has been obtained, then every 6 months is good preventive medicine.

THE CREATIVE RESTORATION DIET

This message is specifically for you! This is a health program designed for modern living with a great deal of study and practical clinical experience to back it up. Any program can only be as effective as its application. Anything worth doing is worth doing well. So why not make it a real challenge to put it to work for a mere 30 days of your life and, in return, have a chance at increased health, the greatest achievement of all.

INCOMPATIBLE WITH THIS PROGRAM

Certain habits are incompatible with your search for health. You cannot build with one hand while tearing down with the other and expect to fashion a monument. The following are incompatible with good health:

1. **Consumption of alcohol.** This has been proven scientifically to destroy brain as well as liver cells.

2. **Smoking.** So much evidence has been presented that we need not elaborate, but specifically, it is carcinogenic and destroys Vitamin C.

3. **Over-consumption of coffee or tea.** Both of these contain habit-forming drugs and are deleterious to the central nervous system. You may substitute herb teas and cereal beverages (see your local health food stores).

UNDERSTANDING THE
CREATIVE RESTORATION DIET

This is a recommended method of eating foods to induce you to "automatically" improve your diet. IT MUST BE UNDERSTOOD, not just blindly followed. You must learn to lead your own way. Unlike the dull, restricted menu-type diet which requires discipline to enforce, this educational approach can be interesting. It encourages a greater rather than lesser variety of foods, thus both taste and appetite are more likely to be satisfied. There is also a great satisfaction in being able to select foods by reason of good judgement and common sense, rather than by the usual hit or miss method.

Therefore, please read the following information carefully. If you understand why you are asked to follow certain rules and guidelines, it will be much easier to gain your cooperation. It merely takes plain, common sense and a wisp of will power. Your conscience should become your guide. Since this diet consists primarily of vegetables, it is high in minerals, especially potassium, which is an essential mineral of prime importance in the body chemistry. Because it is high in fiber foods, which are both cleansing and speed up the tract time, it encourages a favorable intestinal environment. It is intended to eliminate a high proportion of so-called "empty calorie" foods, so it should have an excellent **weight normalization** influence.

Naturally all of the foods which one should not eat cannot be mentioned. Only the major classifications are mentioned in this regard, listing a few categories only. The guidelines for food combinations are few and easy to follow. Emphasis is placed upon the positive "what to eat" nature of dieting. It is a diet you can believe in because it is deemed to be right, founded in truth rather than fancy or statistics. **Basic rules to follow are listed at the end of the text. These should be learned and practiced until they become matters of habit.**

GENERAL PRINCIPLES

Regarding White Flour and White Sugar Products - Not only are white flour and sugar products devoid of their natural occurring vitamins and minerals, but the less desirable calories are concentrated until they become little more than pure starch and carbohydrate. Why is this abuse of Nature's stores brought about.

In the case of white flour, life is the main reason. All commercial white flour is processed so that it can be stored for long periods of time. To make this possible, most of the "life" is removed from the whole wheat berries. Since the oil is removed, it cannot turn rancid.

Everything subject to oxidation has been removed. If it were not so, spoilage would be very rapid. often within a period of a few days.

White sugar is refined for another reason. In its liquid form as can juice, it would ferment rapidly and would require refrigeration from cane field to user. Obviously this would not serve commercial purposes. Granulated sugar did! But, the attendant loss of vitamins and minerals, plus the intensive concentration of purified carbohydrates, makes the mixture too rich to handle by your body, much like the carburetor on you car when too much gas is mixed with the air.

An important feature of the Creative Restoration Diet is to **eat maximum quantities of live foods and eliminate purified foods**. White flour products and white sugar products are dead foods (no enzymes and most or all of the vitamins and minerals removed) and are purified substances which the body finds difficult to adapt to normal metabolism.

It is comparatively simple to eliminate much white sugar from the diet simply by not eating candy, pastries and so forth made of white sugar. However, many find it difficult to eliminate all white flour products such as bread, bakery rolls, paste foods (macaroni, spaghetti, pizza and the like). However, the elimination of white flour products is essential if the fullest benefits are to be obtained from the Creative Restoration Diet.

Regarding the Use of Uncooked Foods - Let's look at your diet from the aspect of how much of it consists of uncooked or raw foods. Many people eat little raw food other than a smattering of lettuce or an occasional glass of fruit juice. The remainder of their diet is completely cooked! **The eating of fresh, raw foods daily should never be let to chance.** Two outstanding all-season foods are recommended as always being available:

1. Tomatoes and Tomato Juice
2. Raw Cabbage

Although raw tomatoes are usually best, canned tomatoes without preservatives added are on the list of acceptable foods. Tomatoes are one of the few vegetables which lend themselves well to the canning process. In fact, because tomatoes are canned at the height of their natural perfection, the food value can be higher than the hot-house varieties sold in off-seasons. The same applies to tomato juice, with both offering rich sources of potassium and Vitamins A, B and C.

Salads made with raw cabbage instead of lettuce can be one of the greatest taste surprises you have ever had. Cabbage in raw form is one of our richest sources of essential vitamins and minerals. It stores well if not better than any other raw food, keeping its nutrients beneath its protective wrapper in the leaves. **It is indispensable to the success of this diet that a high-quality raw food be included in the diet daily.** Tomatoes and cabbage have been suggested. If at all possible, I use one cupful of raw cabbage with a little raw potato or jicama or water chestnuts mixed in every day. Raw carrots, cauliflower, sprouts, celery, etc., are almost always available and can be used to excellent advantage.

Regarding the Use of Meat Products - Meats such as veal, beef, lamb and chicken are good sources of protein. However, even though the protein intake is adequate insofar as quantity is concerned, quality is an even more important point to consider. Incomplete proteins leave out pieces of the "building block" mechanism and, like jigsaw puzzle with pieces missing, the whole picture suffers. This can be a good reason to supplement the diet with a multi-source protein product to assure an adequate amino acid supply and balance.

Also in regard to protein ingestion, its breakdown into amino acids is essential to its utilization. This is called the process of digestion. If digestion fails to liquefy the meat (protein), spoilage can occur in the intestinal tract - a process called putrefaction. Effects of putrefaction in the gastrointestinal tract are bad breath, foul-odored stool and a general decrease in energy. This is good reason to supplement the diet with an appropriate digestive enzyme product, both facilitating breakdown of the protein and preventing putrefaction.

Contrary to some opinions, the grinding of meat into small particles, e.g. hamburger, does not increase its digestibility. One the other hand, grinding of meat can have deleterious effects. Ground meat spoils rapidly at room temperature, whole meat does not. In fact, aging of whole meat can make it more tender by a sort of "predigestion" which occurs.

It is postulated that nucleic acids are released when meat is ground, coming out with the meat juices apparently making spoilage very fast by this means. Similar action may occur when ground meat is introduced into the intestinal tract. There the temperature is ideal for rapid spoilage. **This is particularly applicable if there is insufficient hydrochloric acid in the stomach**, as HCl acts as an intestinal anti-septic to inhibit fermentation and putrefaction which might otherwise occur. Here again, a proper digestive aid containing hydrochloric acid sources may be used to a distinct advantage.

NOTE: Preserved meats such as wieners and sausages do not have as much tendency to putrefaction since they contain anti-putrefactive chemicals (usually nitrites and/or nitrates) which work both inside and outside the body to produce this effect. However, for the same reason, they are not desirable from a nutritional viewpoint. It has been determined that these substances inhibit enzymes in the body, produce liver and kidney diseases as well as being possibly carcinogenic.

Regarding the Use of Sugar and Protein and/or Fat Combinations. - One of the little known deleterious effects of refined sugar is its reaction in the gastrointestinal tract with protein and/or fat combinations. First of all, let us establish that concentrated carbohydrates (sugars) stay in the stomach for only a short period of time since very little digestion is necessary. On the other hand, protein remains in the stomach for extended periods of time (up to 5 hours) because much activity must take place before the proteins can be passed on to the small intestine for absorption. Some fats also are broken down in the stomach and the presence of fat in the stomach slows down the production of hydrochloric acid which further delays the time of departure of stomach contents. When concentrated carbohydrates are mixed with protein or protein/fat combinations, sugars tend to ferment in the stomach producing gas. Adequate hydrochloric acid will prevent this to some extent, but the major cause of stomach gas is improper combining of food groups. Too many Americans are accustomed to finishing off a good protein meal with sweet desserts. For best nutrient, concentrated sweets should be eaten on an empty stomach. This includes fruits, fruit juices, etc., as well.

There are many sugar/protein combinations which may be easily avoided if one is on the alert. An outstanding example is eggs with orange juice. The fact that many foods contain a combination of protein and carbohydrate must be taken into consideration. Such natural combinations rarely give much trouble as it is the concentration of carbohydrate which produce the deleterious effects; these being proportional to the quantity present.

Regarding the Use of Fiber Foods in the Diet - As a natural laxative with griping, diarrhea or any of the other complaints we have about other laxatives, dietary fiber has no equal. Although many are not aware, they may suffer from extremely slow movement of the digestive tract. There are many consequences of such slow tract time.

Intestinal gas because of the fermentation of starches and sugar.

Diverticulosis due to the large amounts of fecal material pushing against the wall of the intestine, producing little sacs or pouches which then fill with waste material. This is an ideal circumstance for more putrefaction to occur which then discharges noxious matter into the tract which may be absorbed into the blood stream.

Hemorrhoids and varicostities can be blamed at least in part to the pressure exerted by the large amounts of material collects in the intestinal tract on the pelvic veins creating back pressure which balloons the veins in the hemorrhoidal plexus and in the leg.

THE FOOD COMMANDMENTS

Thou shalt eat one bowl of whole grain cereal daily, single or multiple grains, hot or cold.

Thou shalt eat four cupfuls of vegetables daily, cooked or raw, but some of each, preferably half and half.

Thou shalt eat one cup of whole fruit daily.

Thou shalt never eat margarine, shortening or unsaturated oils as they depress the immune system and hasten your demise.

Thou shalt use butter, olive oil and peanut oil as the concentrated fat in your diet.

Thou shalt consume a variety of fish, fowl and meats if desired; dairy products, nuts and seeds. Eggs are good food. All of these are in addition, not in place of the four cupfuls of vegetables, one cup of fruit and one bowl of cereal daily.

Regarding the Use of Common Salt in the Diet - People who use as much salt as they like may excrete 9 times as much potassium, an essential minerals, as those on salt-restricted diets. Actually, Americans frequently consume 20 to 25 times as much salt as estimated sodium requirements recommend. If this is not counter-balanced with increased potassium intake, a borderline potassium deficiency state is easily brought about. Salt substitutes, mostly made up of potassium chloride, are often too bitter for anyone to stick with. We are fortunate in having a new 40-60 mixture of sodium and potassium chlorides on the market. This satisfies flavor requirements and you need not worry about the loss of potassium from using sodium chloride alone. This formula is available in most supermarkets and health food stores.

Many form of chronic degenerative diseases are initially caused by the body's reaction to specific micro-organisms we call KLEPTIC MICROBES. This text dealt with one manifestation of this infection:

ARTHRITIS

The AL-DON INSTITUTE OF EXPERIMENTAL MEDICINE has developed a specific vaccine for these microbes.

This document covered the history of the discovery of the Kleptic Microbe, the development of hormonal, nutritional and specific vaccine therapies.

Microbes are best observed through a darkfield microscope. The following diagram shows the microscope looking at the content of a drop (greatly enlarged) of blood.

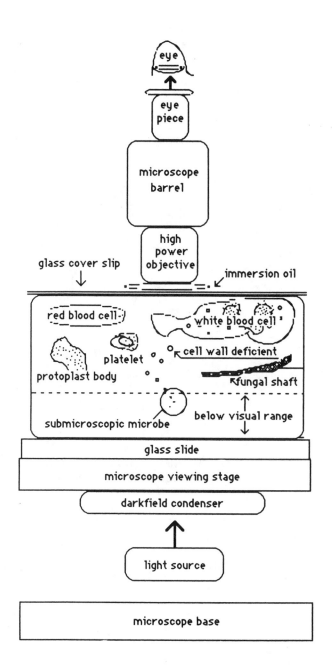

eye

eye piece

microscope barrel

high power objective

glass cover slip

immersion oil

red blood cell

white blood cell

cell wall deficient

platelet

protoplast body

fungal shaft

submicroscopic microbe

below visual range

glass slide

microscope viewing stage

darkfield condenser

light source

microscope base

We will now take the part of the above diagram that is in the "below visual range" and enlarge it.

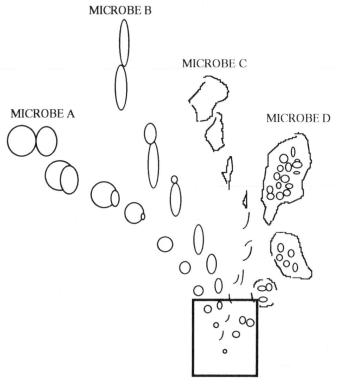

MICROBE B

MICROBE C

MICROBE A

MICROBE D

WITHIN THE BOX ARE MICROBES
BELOW LIGHT-MICROSCOPE RESOLUTION
AND THEREFORE INVISIBLE

In discussing the Kleptic Microbes, we are most concerned with what lives below the visual range of the bright-field microscope.

In the example diagram above A, B, C and D are listed. These might represent life forms that have been observed, studied and labeled by researchers only because they were visible. But what about the ones that were not observed, not studied and not labeled? Do these entities simply not exist? If they do exist, what are they and what do they do?

What is the relationship between the progenitors of A and B, or B and C, C and D, or A and D and so on? As an analogy, the present scientific establishments are looking at the airplane, the tank, the bullet and the bomb. We are looking at the iron from which all were made and the developmental steps that lead up to what is called the final product. But, what happens when the airplanes, bullets, bombs, etc., are dismantled and recycled to become refrigerators, radios and wrist watches? Is there a relationship between one and the other?

The establishment's present philosophy is to develop defenses and countermeasures for the finished product. That's only effective after the war starts. Wouldn't it be better to just stop sending the enemy the steel necessary to build their weapons in the first place? Our approach is to strike at the root, not just the flower. If we are fighting a deadly microbe, wouldn't we be more successful dealing with it before it becomes deadly?

SUMMARY

Arthritis is a significant example of the many factors which produce a breakdown of what should be a marvelously functioning body. It is not due to a single cause, but is the result of many changes in normal function. To restore normalcy, as many as possible of these abnormal factors must be addressed. When such is implemented, remarkable changes for the better occur in a relatively short period of time. The compounded experience of the two authors has resulted in a protocol that offers phenomenal results. Here are the major steps:

1. The institution of a detoxification process utilizing:
    a. A 3-day controlled fast;
    b. Superoxygenation of the body orally, intra-venously and rectally.

2. Intensive and significant supplemental nutrient support.

3. Use of Ion Extractor Therapy to remove toxic metals and increase circulation.

4. Balancing of hormones through the use of carefully controlled sublingual micro-doses of tissue rebuilding hormones.

5. Depletion or deletion of colonies of the Kleptic Microbe by special infusions.

6. The application of Immune Modulating Blueprint

injections to prevent re-infestation by the Kleptic Microbes.

7. The adherence to a common sense way of eating designed to give the most benefit with the greatest latitude in food choice.